SAVE YOUR EDGES

Workbook

SAVE YOUR EDGES
Workbook

Written by Brianna Laren
Artwork by Delmaine Donson

Copyright © 2021 by Brianna Laren
Illustrator: Delmaine Donson

All rights reserved, including the right to reproduce this book or portions thereof in any form whatsoever. No part of this publication may be reproduced, distributed, or transmitted in any form or by any means, including photocopying, recording, or other electronic or mechanical methods, without the prior written permission of the publisher, except in the case of brief quotations embodied in critical reviews and certain other noncommercial uses permitted by copyright law.

For information about special discounts for bulk purchases, please contact us at info@BriannaLaren.com.
www.BriannaLaren.com

Printed in the United States of America

ISBN: 978-0-578-33005-1
(Paperback)

This book is dedicated to those who forgot to love themselves first and need a reminder that they are worthy of all the beautiful things they pour into others.

In Loving Memory of:
Brooks Shands

More books by this author:
Breebe's Brand New Baby Brother
Pretty Pretty Black Girl
Edge Control for the Soul

-- from the book Edge Control for the Soul

save your edges by brianna laren

so many women out here
are broken to pieces
because they are trying to make
some man do right by them
& i'm not judging because i've been there
but here is a tip that will
save you a lot of time and therapy

stop sacrificing your

sanity
joy
time
edges
youth
money
credibility
self esteem
self worth

your ---> self

all for people
who don't care enough about you
to not make you sacrifice
those things in the first place

and that goes for everyone
not just some man
but anyone and everyone
save your edges baby

Contents

Self Love

This is where it all begins, where you set the bar. How you love yourself will be reflected in your relationships, friendships, and your daily life.

Mental Health

If your mental health is suffering, it will seep into other areas of your life and you won't have any edges to save. Take this time to get your mind right. Identify your trauma & your triggers, set healthy boundaries and map out your steps to heal.

Dreams + Goals

Life hits different when you know where you want to go and how to get there. It doesn't mean you won't hit bumps in the road or get lost along the way, it just means you can readjust and get back on track. That's why it is important to know what you want & set goals to get it.

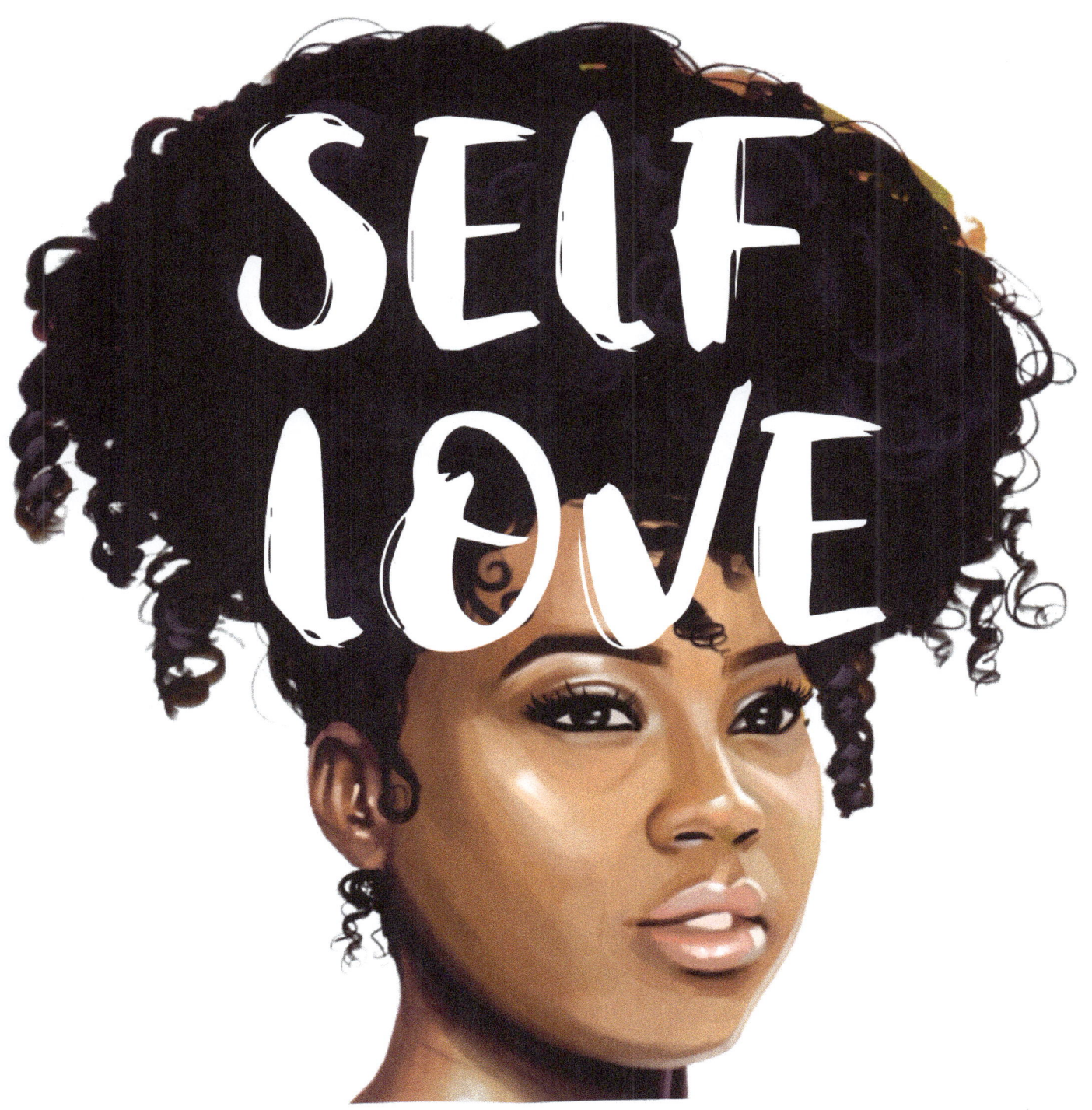

Self love is deep conditioner for your soul. It nurtures, moisturizes, & maintains what is within you and it's the first step to saving your edges. Do you remember the time it took to learn your hair type, what products made your curls pop, how to avoid frizz, which protective styles give you definition versus volume? Let's take that same process and apply it to getting to know ourselves. It's all trial and error really which takes time but the best part is seeing the growth after you've put in the work.

my self love goals:

SOME PEOPLE WILL NEVER ROOT FOR YOU & THAT'S OKAY

#SAVEYOUREDGES

one thing i love about myself:
___

why i love this about myself:
___

an area in my life i can improve:
_____
_____
_____
_____
_____
_____
_____
_____
_____
_____
_____
_____
_____
_____

ways to improve this area of my life:
_____
_____
_____
_____
_____
_____
_____
_____
_____
_____
_____
_____

how i celebrate myself:
_____
_____
_____
_____
_____
_____
_____
_____
_____
_____
_____
_____

how i want to celebrate myself:
_____
_____
_____
_____
_____
_____
_____
_____
_____
_____
_____
_____

how can i be intentional about celebrating myself?
_____
_____
_____
_____
_____
_____
_____
_____
_____
_____
_____
_____
_____
_____
_____

how do i want others to celebrate me?
_____
_____
_____
_____
_____
_____
_____
_____
_____
_____
_____
_____
_____

SPEAK TO YOURSELF LIKE A BEST FRIEND INSTEAD OF LIKE YOUR WORST CRITIC. BE KIND, GENTLE, AFFIRMING, & MOST OF ALL LOVING. YOU DESERVE GRACE.

#SAVEYOUREDGES

some recent wins (big and small):
___

some recent wins (big and small):

how i see myself:

how i can improve my self image:

how i can stop negative self talk:

negative things i think/say about myself:
___

turn them into positive statements:
___

YOUR WORDS HOLD POWER. USE THEM WISELY.

#SAVEYOUREDGES

affirmations i can speak to myself daily:

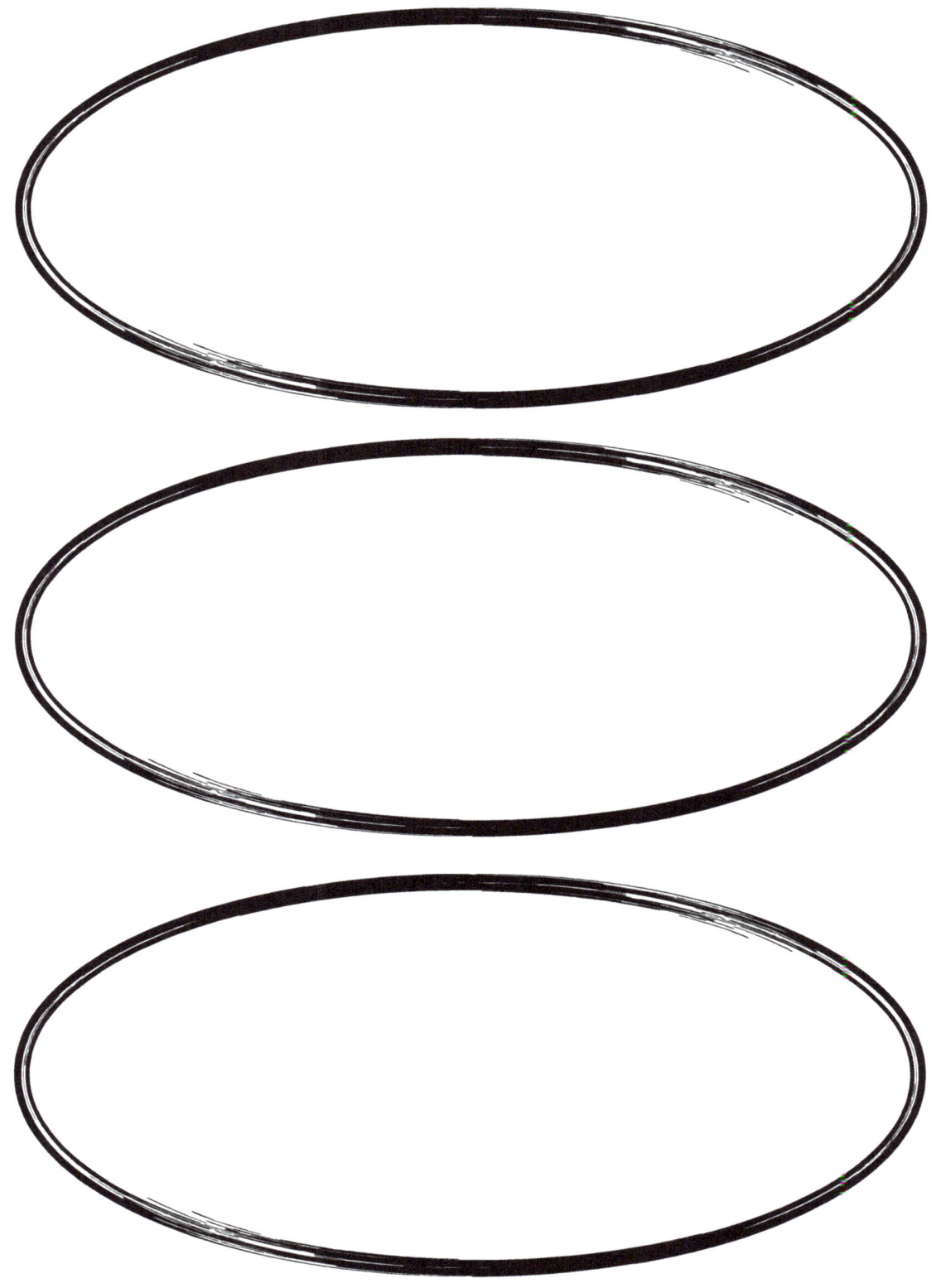

how these affirmations make me feel:
___

how i can incorporate these into my day:
___

five things i love about myself:

___

why i love these things about myself:

___

how can i be kind to myself today?

how can i make this a habit?

how can i stand up for myself today?

how can i make this a habit?

I'VE LEARNED TO VALUE FRIENDSHIPS THAT HAVE WEATHERED STORMS OVER THOSE THAT CRUMBLED AT THE FIRST SIGN OF RAIN

#SAVEYOUREDGES

my circle of friends include:
_____
_____
_____
_____
_____
_____
_____
_____
_____
_____
_____
_____
_____

what i love about my circle:
_____
_____
_____
_____
_____
_____
_____
_____
_____
_____
_____
_____
_____

how important is friendship to me?

what i've learned about friendship:

how i can pour into my friends:

_____
_____
_____
_____
_____
_____
_____
_____
_____
_____
_____
_____
_____
_____

how my friends can pour into me:

_____
_____
_____
_____
_____
_____
_____
_____
_____
_____
_____
_____
_____
_____

ten things i love about myself:
___

why i love these things about myself:
___

an area in my life i want to improve:
_____
_____
_____
_____
_____
_____
_____
_____
_____
_____
_____
_____
_____
_____

how improving this will impact my life:
_____
_____
_____
_____
_____
_____
_____
_____
_____
_____
_____
_____
_____
_____

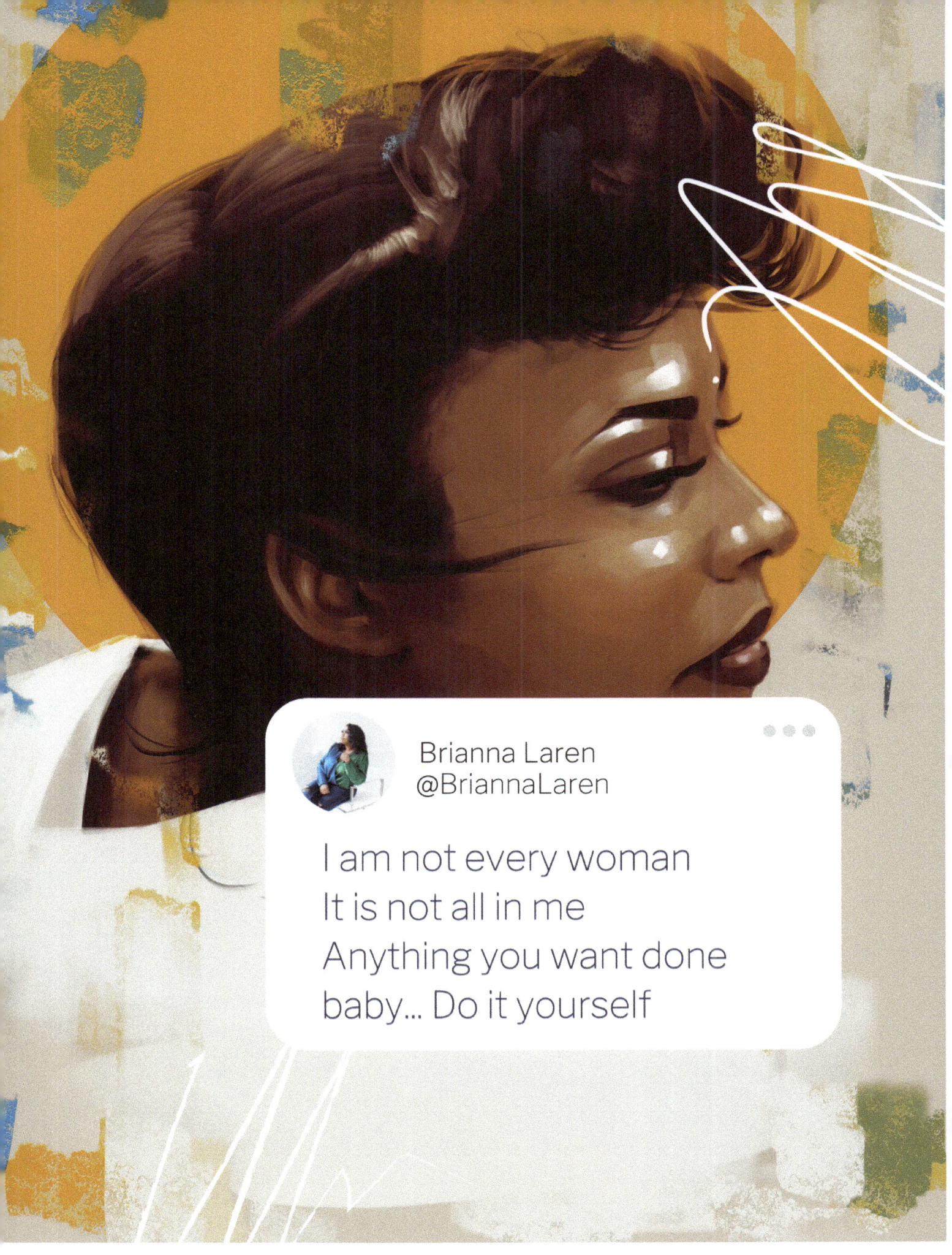

what makes me smile?

what fills me with joy?

things that makes me laugh:
_____
_____
_____
_____
_____
_____
_____
_____
_____
_____
_____
_____
_____
_____

my favorite scents:
_____
_____
_____
_____
_____
_____
_____
_____
_____
_____
_____
_____

my favorite movies:
_____
_____
_____
_____
_____
_____
_____
_____
_____
_____
_____
_____

my favorite tv shows:
_____
_____
_____
_____
_____
_____
_____
_____
_____
_____
_____
_____

my hidden talent:
___

how i discovered this talent:
___

my deepest fear:
___

what tools can i use to overcome it?
___

WE GIVE OUR JOY AWAY IN THE SMALLEST OF WAYS... LIKE CHOOSING SILENCE OVER SPEAKING UP FOR OURSELVES TO MAKE OTHERS COMFORTABLE. LET THEM BE UNCOMFORTABLE SIS

#SAVEYOUREDGES

fifteen things i love about myself:
_____
_____
_____
_____
_____
_____
_____
_____
_____
_____
_____
_____
_____
_____
_____

why i love these things about myself:
_____
_____
_____
_____
_____
_____
_____
_____
_____
_____
_____
_____
_____
_____

my favorite foods:
_____
_____
_____
_____
_____
_____
_____
_____
_____
_____
_____
_____
_____

my favorite people to talk to:
_____
_____
_____
_____
_____
_____
_____
_____
_____
_____
_____
_____

my go-to dance move:
___

when/how did i learn this move?

my favorite childhood memory:
_____
_____
_____
_____
_____
_____
_____
_____
_____
_____
_____
_____
_____
_____
_____
_____
_____
_____
_____
_____
_____
_____
_____
_____
_____
_____
_____

what i love about this memory:

I AM HAPPY WITH THE PERSON ♡ I AM BECOMING

#SAVEYOUREDGES

my favorite recent memory:

what i love about this memory:

10+ songs i'd put on an uplifting playlist:

my fave feel good song lyrics:

what are my gifts?

_____
_____
_____
_____
_____
_____
_____
_____
_____
_____
_____
_____
_____
_____

how can i use them?

_____
_____
_____
_____
_____
_____
_____
_____
_____
_____
_____
_____
_____
_____

what keeps me grounded?

I HOPE YOU KNOW
HOW
LOVED
YOU
ARE
#SAVEYOUREDGES

when do i feel the most loved?

what is my love language?

how can i practice that language on myself?

something i am looking forward to:

a place i look forward to visiting one day:

how can i show myself grace daily?

a love letter to myself:

I LOVE MYSELF MORE EACH DAY

#SAVEYOUREDGES

key takeaways from this section:

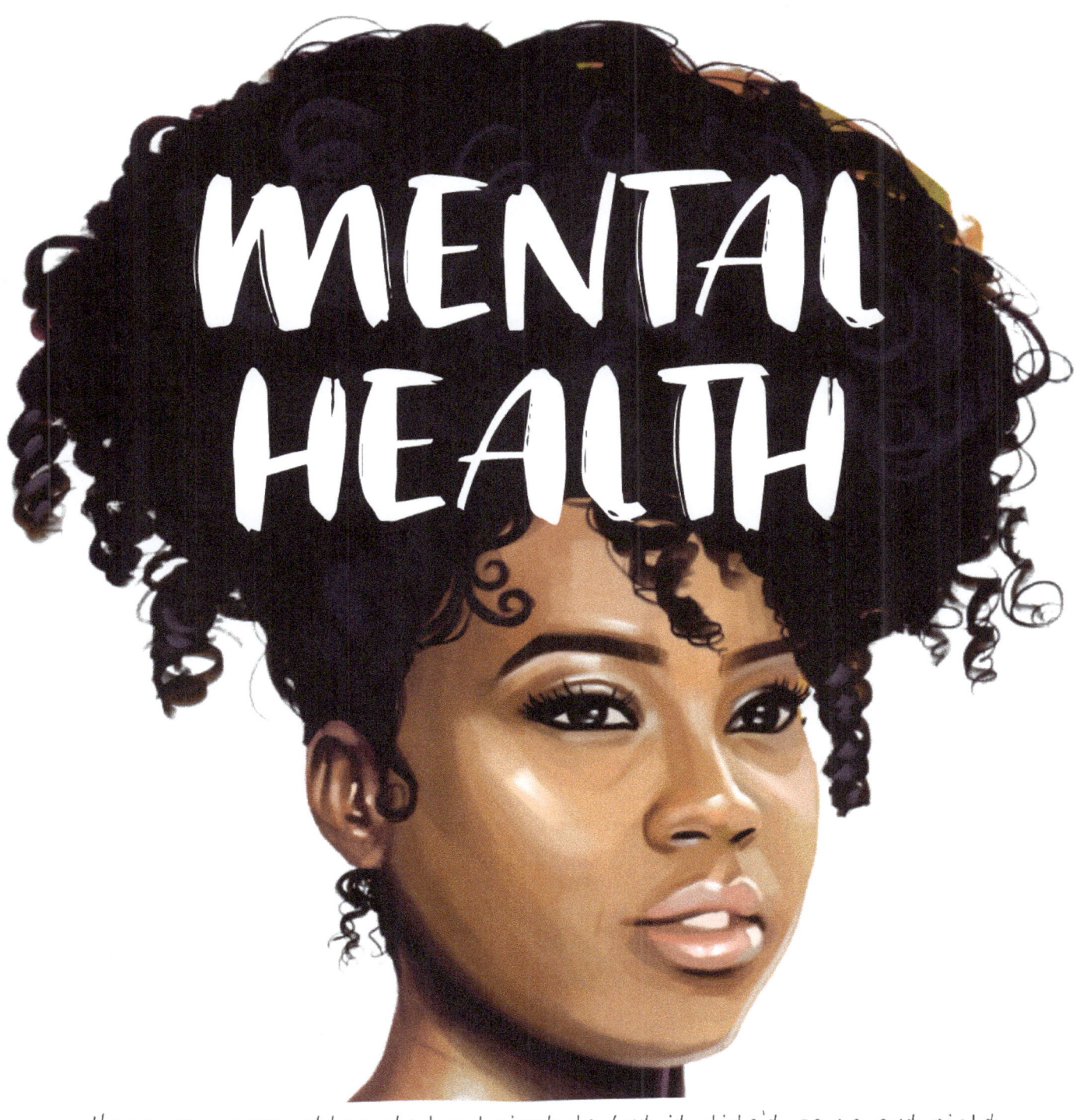

MENTAL HEALTH

Have you ever attempted a hairstyle but it didn't come out right because you needed a trim? The truth is it doesn't matter how hard you try if your ends are split, tore up, and raggedy the style is going to suffer. It is tough to hide damage and it is the same way in life. I don't care how good you look, how beat your face is, how funny, kind, or fashionable you are... it will all be in vain if your mental health is in shambles. Take this time to heal, sis. This is your safe space.

mental health goals:

IT'S OKAY TO PRIORITIZE YOUR MENTAL HEALTH

#SAVEYOUREDGES

how can i prioritize my health?

how can i prioritize my peace?

how can i prioritize my mental health?

how can i make this a habit?

how can i get more in tune with myself?

how can i listen to myself more?

how will these changes impact my life?

what calms/relaxes me?

_____
_____
_____
_____
_____
_____
_____
_____
_____
_____
_____
_____
_____
_____

calming activities i can add to my routine:

_____
_____
_____
_____
_____
_____
_____
_____
_____
_____
_____
_____

how can i be more present in the moment?

Dear Black Woman,

You do not have to be strong every second of every day. You are allowed to fall apart. You are allowed to come undone. You are allowed to ask for help. You are allowed to take time to put yourself back together. You do not need permission to be human.

#saveyouredges

how can i make more time for myself?
___

how do i feel when i make time for myself?
___

how feeling overwhelmed affects my life:
_____
_____
_____
_____
_____
_____
_____
_____
_____
_____
_____
_____
_____
_____

ways i can prevent becoming overwhelmed:
_____
_____
_____
_____
_____
_____
_____
_____
_____
_____
_____
_____
_____
_____

what makes me feel safe?

_____
_____
_____
_____
_____
_____
_____
_____
_____
_____
_____
_____
_____
_____

what makes me feel comfortable?

_____
_____
_____
_____
_____
_____
_____
_____
_____
_____
_____
_____

what makes me trust someone?

___

who do i feel safe around?

___

what makes me put my guard up?

_____

where does this stem from?

_____

YOU DON'T HAVE TO DO IT ALONE ALL OF THE TIME... IT'S OKAY TO ASK FOR HELP

#SAVEYOUREDGES

am i good at asking for help? why/why not

how do i feel when i ask for help?

how i can improve my perception of help:
___

one thing i can ask for help with today:
___

what is my trauma?

how does it make me feel?

how trauma affects my life:

NO MORE TRAUMA OR WHATEVER MARY J SAID...

#SAVEYOUREDGES

what am i doing to address the trauma?

steps to overcome the trauma

steps to overcome the trauma

what are my triggers?

what caused my triggers:

YOU DESERVE TO HEAL

#SAVEYOUREDGES

how to identify when i'm triggered:

healthy ways to cope:

a situation i thought i wouldn't overcome but did:
_____
_____
_____
_____
_____
_____
_____
_____
_____
_____
_____
_____
_____
_____
_____
_____
_____
_____
_____
_____
_____
_____
_____
_____
_____
_____
_____
_____

how i overcame it & how i felt afterwards:

ways to give myself grace & time to heal:

SOMETIMES THE HARDEST PERSON TO FORGIVE IS YOURSELF...

#SAVEYOUREDGES

something i need to forgive myself for:
___

how i can forgive myself and move forward:
___

why it's important to forgive myself:

_____
_____
_____
_____
_____
_____
_____
_____
_____
_____
_____
_____
_____
_____
_____

how i feel after forgiving myself:

_____
_____
_____
_____
_____
_____
_____
_____
_____
_____
_____
_____
_____
_____

something i need to forgive someone else for:
___

how i can forgive them and move forward:
___

healthy ways to communicate with others about how their actions/words affect me:

how do i react to challenges?

IT IS OKAY TO RESTRICT ACCESS TO CERTAIN PEOPLE IN ORDER TO PROTECT YOUR PEACE

#SAVEYOUREDGES

lessons from recent challenges:
_____
_____
_____
_____
_____
_____
_____
_____
_____
_____
_____
_____
_____
_____

how i can handle difficult situations better:
_____
_____
_____
_____
_____
_____
_____
_____
_____
_____
_____
_____

how do i handle disappointment?

why do i react this way?

_____

do i need to improve? If so, what/how?

_____

how do i handle criticism?

why do i react this way?

do i need to improve? If so, what/how?

Some people don't want you to heal because they don't want to be inconvenienced by your boundaries. -Heal anyway-
#saveyouredges

how do i handle uncertainty?

is it productive? If not, how can it be?

how i take responsibility for my actions:

_____
_____
_____
_____
_____
_____
_____
_____
_____
_____
_____
_____
_____
_____

how can i hold myself accountable?

_____
_____
_____
_____
_____
_____
_____
_____
_____
_____
_____
_____

one healthy boundary i can set today:
boundaries can be mental, emotional, physical, financial, or energy/time

_____
_____
_____
_____
_____
_____
_____
_____
_____
_____
_____
_____

how will i enforce this boundary?

_____
_____
_____
_____
_____
_____
_____
_____
_____
_____
_____
_____

how setting boundaries will impact me:
_____
_____
_____
_____
_____
_____
_____
_____
_____
_____
_____
_____
_____
_____

how i can make this a habit:
_____
_____
_____
_____
_____
_____
_____
_____
_____
_____
_____
_____
_____

who i have problems setting boundaries with:
_____
_____
_____
_____
_____
_____
_____
_____
_____
_____
_____
_____
_____
_____

how i can move past that & set boundaries:
_____
_____
_____
_____
_____
_____
_____
_____
_____
_____
_____
_____

5 boundaries i can set:

_____
_____
_____
_____
_____
_____
_____
_____
_____
_____
_____
_____
_____
_____

how i will enforce them:

_____
_____
_____
_____
_____
_____
_____
_____
_____
_____
_____
_____
_____
_____

Give yourself permission to pause. There is beauty in stillness. There is healing in silence. Rest. Relax. Recover. Repeat.

#saveyouredges

one boundary i set & enforced this week:

how enforcing made me feel:
_____
_____
_____
_____
_____
_____
_____
_____
_____
_____
_____
_____
_____
_____

how this boundary will help me:
_____
_____
_____
_____
_____
_____
_____
_____
_____
_____

two boundaries i set & enforced this month:

how enforcing made me feel:
_____
_____
_____
_____
_____
_____
_____
_____
_____
_____
_____
_____
_____

how these boundaries will help me:
_____
_____
_____
_____
_____
_____
_____
_____
_____
_____
_____

NO THANK YOU.
NO THANKS.
NOPE.
NO.
ARE ALL COMPLETE SENTENCES

#SAVEYOUREDGES

how do i feel today?

how can i think positively today?

_____

how can i make a "bad day" better?

_____

how can i acknowledge my feelings daily?

ways i can check in with myself daily:

I AM IN CHARGE OF HOW I FEEL AND TODAY I CHOOSE JOY

#SAVEYOUREDGES

what is going on in my life right now?

how am i showing up for myself?

_____
_____
_____
_____
_____
_____
_____
_____
_____
_____
_____
_____
_____
_____

how can i show up for myself consistently?

_____
_____
_____
_____
_____
_____
_____
_____
_____
_____
_____
_____

what is going well in my life right now?

how can i apply this to other areas of my life?

what i want to be going better:

how i can improve this area:

ANXIETY, DEPRESSION, IMPOSTER SYNDROME WILL NOT WIN TODAY. YOU WILL WIN TODAY!

#SAVEYOUREDGES

what/where is my safe space?

_____
_____
_____
_____
_____
_____
_____
_____
_____
_____
_____
_____

what makes it feel safe?

_____
_____
_____
_____
_____
_____
_____
_____
_____
_____

ways i can decompress:
_____
_____
_____
_____
_____
_____
_____
_____
_____
_____
_____
_____
_____
_____
_____

ways i can get out of a bad mood:
_____
_____
_____
_____
_____
_____
_____
_____
_____
_____
_____
_____
_____

my fave feel good quotes:

how gratitude can change the way i view life:

ten things i am grateful for:

people i am grateful for:
_____
_____
_____
_____
_____
_____
_____
_____
_____
_____
_____
_____
_____

lessons i learned from them:
_____
_____
_____
_____
_____
_____
_____
_____
_____
_____
_____
_____

I HAVE ENOUGH
I DO ENOUGH
I AM ENOUGH

#SAVEYOUREDGES

key takeaways from this section:

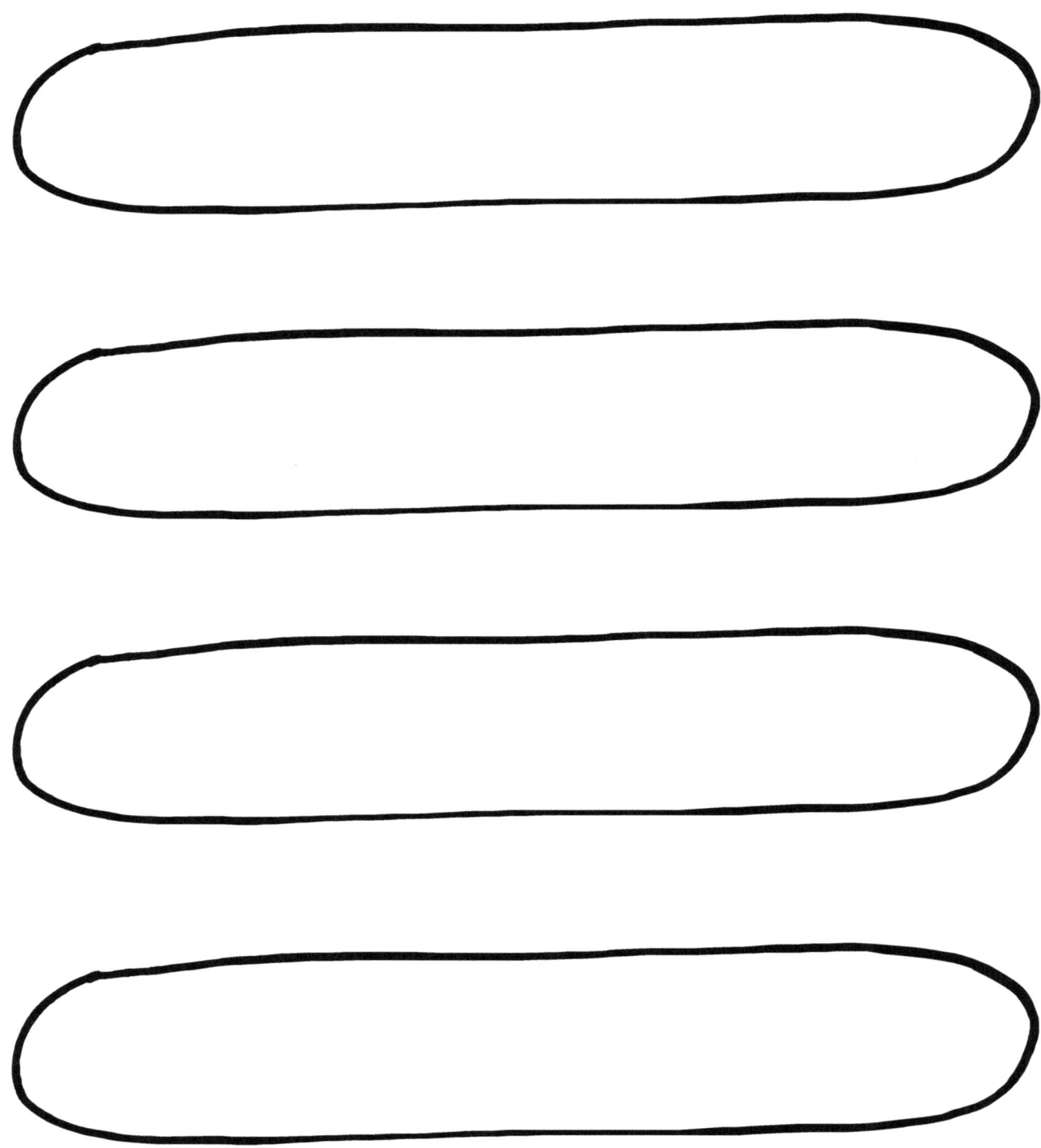

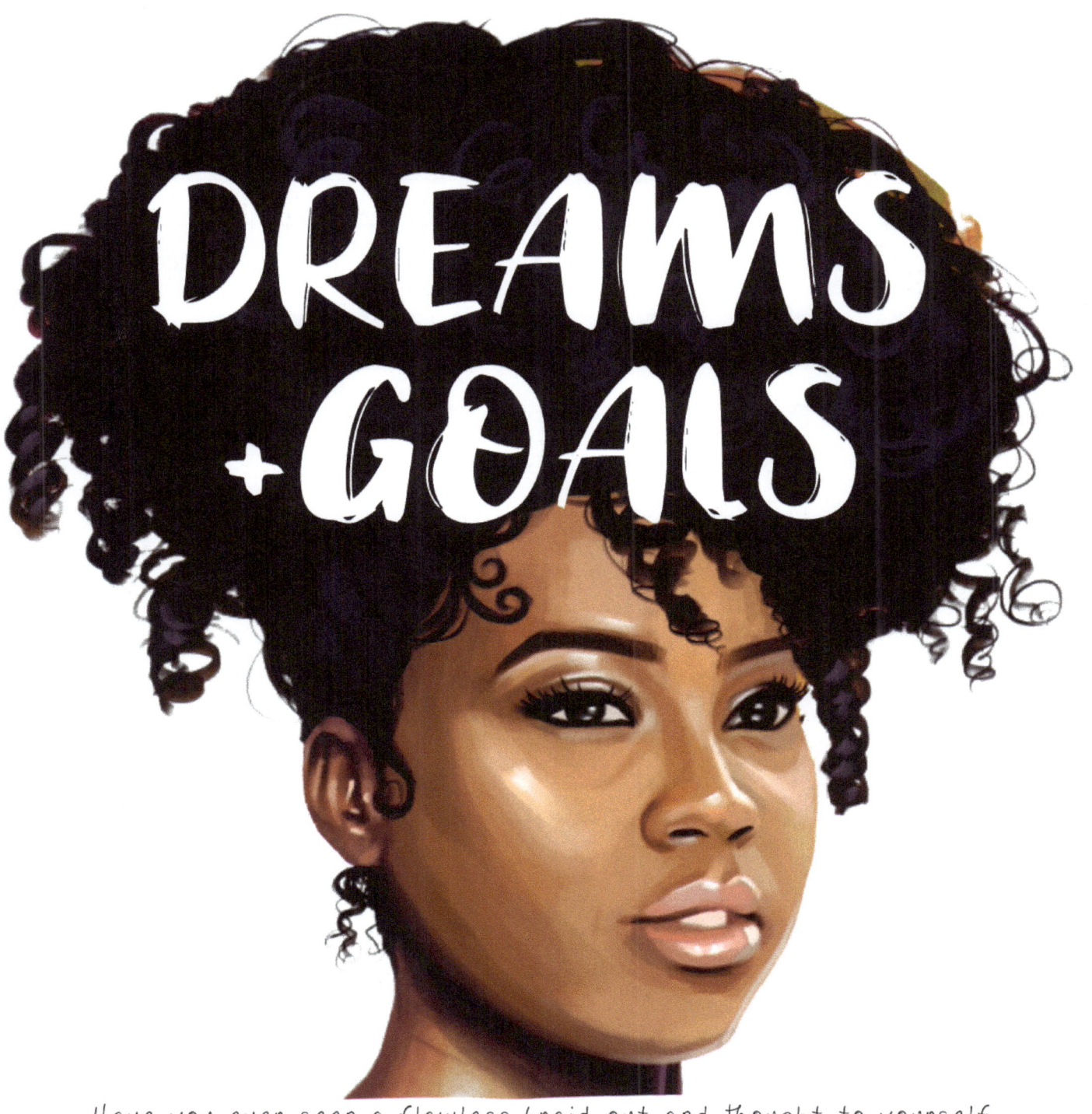

DREAMS + GOALS

Have you ever seen a flawless braid out and thought to yourself #hairgoals? I know I have. Sometimes it's pure luck that their hair turned out that way or maybe even genetics but most times it's because they had a strategy. They planned out what products & technique to use, dry time, tools needed, & possibly even watched a few tutorials first. The point is it took preparation and execution to get the results they wanted. Oddly enough we can use those same tactics to reach our personal goals and dreams.

if i could do anything i would:

_____
_____
_____
_____
_____
_____
_____
_____
_____
_____
_____
_____
_____
_____
_____
_____

what is stopping me?

_____
_____
_____
_____
_____
_____
_____
_____
_____
_____
_____
_____

DREAM BIG

#SAVEYOUREDGES

a belief that is holding me back:

where did this belief come from?

how is it harmful to me reaching my goals?

what is a better alternative to this belief?

my dreams:

what is stopping me?

my plan to bring my dreams to fruition:

my ideal life:

my life goals:

my plan to create ideal life:

my ideal career:

my career goals:

my plan to obtain ideal career:

SURROUND YOURSELF WITH PEOPLE THAT WANT TO POUR INTO YOUR CUP NOT JUST SIP FROM IT

#SAVEYOUREDGES

my ideal friendships:

my friendship goals:

my plan to foster ideal friendships:

my ideal relationship:
___

my relationship goals:

my plan to build ideal relationship:

I AM PLANTING SEEDS THAT WILL BE WATERED AND NURTURED BY FUTURE GENERATIONS

#SAVEYOUREDGES

my ideal family:
family does not always = spouse + children. what does family look like to me?

generational cycles i need to break:

my family goals:

my plan to reach family goals:

my ideal finances:

my financial goals:

my plan to create ideal finances:

budget

bill	due date	amount	needed?
	TOTAL:		

budget

bill	due date	amount	needed?
	TOTAL:		

what can be lowered or cut from my budget?
_____
_____
_____
_____
_____
_____
_____
_____
_____
_____
_____
_____
_____
_____

how this will help reach my financial goals:
_____
_____
_____
_____
_____
_____
_____
_____
_____
_____
_____
_____

What is the point of getting somewhere fast if you are not prepared when you arrive?

#saveyouredges

spending tracker

date	item	amount
	TOTAL:	

spending tracker

date	item	amount

*try to track your spending for 30 days

spending tracker

date	item	amount
	TOTAL:	

spending tracker

date	item	amount
	TOTAL:	

spending tracker

date	item	amount
	TOTAL:	

what i learned about my spending habits:
_____
_____
_____
_____
_____
_____
_____
_____
_____
_____
_____
_____
_____
_____
_____
_____

how my habits can better align w/ my goals:
_____
_____
_____
_____
_____
_____
_____
_____
_____
_____
_____
_____
_____
_____

my ideal home:

i.e. two story home, located in ___, or i want my house to be full of laughter & feel at peace when I walk through the door. more than just material wants.

my home goals:

plan to create my ideal home:

IT'S NOT TOO LATE TO START

(SO GET STARTED)

#SAVEYOUREDGES

how would creating a daily routine benefit me?

monday

wake time

_____

schedule

8:00 _____
9:00 _____
10:00 _____
11:00 _____
12:00 _____
1:00 _____
2:00 _____
3:00 _____
4:00 _____
5:00 _____
6:00 _____
7:00 _____
8:00 _____
9:00 _____
10:00 _____
11:00 _____

affirmation of the day:

tuesday

wake time

_____

schedule

8:00 _____
9:00 _____
10:00 _____
11:00 _____
12:00 _____
1:00 _____
2:00 _____
3:00 _____
4:00 _____
5:00 _____
6:00 _____
7:00 _____
8:00 _____
9:00 _____
10:00 _____
11:00 _____

affirmation of the day:

wednesday

wake time

_____

schedule

8:00 _____
9:00 _____
10:00 _____
11:00 _____
12:00 _____
1:00 _____
2:00 _____
3:00 _____
4:00 _____
5:00 _____
6:00 _____
7:00 _____
8:00 _____
9:00 _____
10:00 _____
11:00 _____

affirmation of the day:

thursday

wake time

_____

schedule

8:00 _____
9:00 _____
10:00 _____
11:00 _____
12:00 _____
1:00 _____
2:00 _____
3:00 _____
4:00 _____
5:00 _____
6:00 _____
7:00 _____
8:00 _____
9:00 _____
10:00 _____
11:00 _____

affirmation of the day:

friday

wake time
_____

schedule

8:00 _____
9:00 _____
10:00 _____
11:00 _____
12:00 _____
1:00 _____
2:00 _____
3:00 _____
4:00 _____
5:00 _____
6:00 _____
7:00 _____
8:00 _____
9:00 _____
10:00 _____
11:00 _____

affirmation of the day:

saturday

wake time
_____

schedule

8:00 _____
9:00 _____
10:00 _____
11:00 _____
12:00 _____
1:00 _____
2:00 _____
3:00 _____
4:00 _____
5:00 _____
6:00 _____
7:00 _____
8:00 _____
9:00 _____
10:00 _____
11:00 _____

affirmation of the day:

sunday

wake time

_____

schedule

8:00 _____
9:00 _____
10:00 _____
11:00 _____
12:00 _____
1:00 _____
2:00 _____
3:00 _____
4:00 _____
5:00 _____
6:00 _____
7:00 _____
8:00 _____
9:00 _____
10:00 _____
11:00 _____

affirmation of the day:

how will these routines help me?
_____
_____
_____
_____
_____
_____
_____
_____
_____
_____
_____

what having a routine will allow me to do:
_____
_____
_____
_____
_____
_____
_____
_____
_____
_____

how can i be more organized?

_____
_____
_____
_____
_____
_____
_____
_____
_____
_____
_____

how will being organized make me feel?

_____
_____
_____
_____
_____
_____
_____
_____
_____
_____
_____

how can i incorporate mindfulness into my day?

Your past is not a reflection of your future. It serves as a reminder of what worked and what did not. Use it to move forward

#SAVEYOUREDGES

key takeaways from this section:

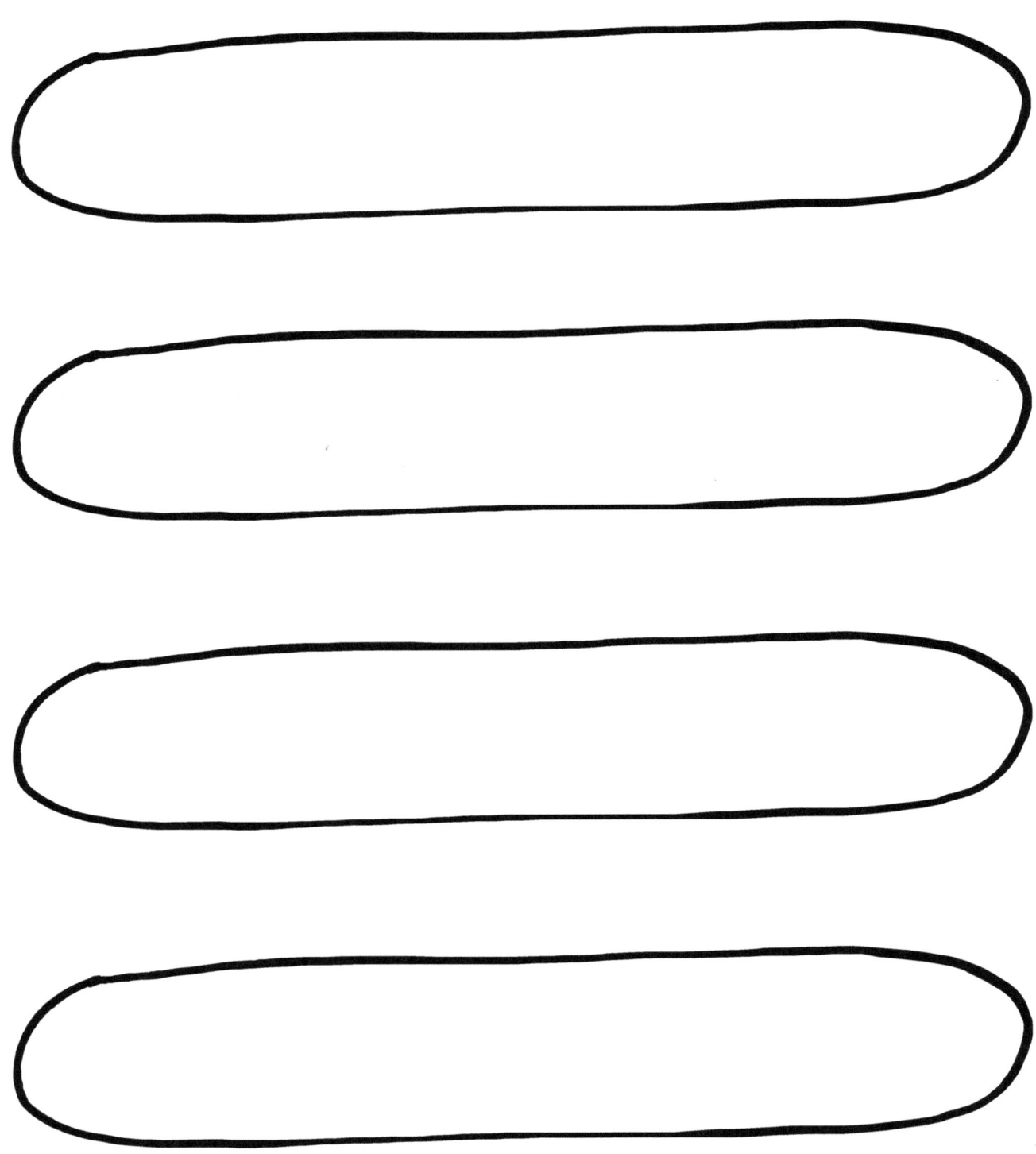

Hey Suga,

You made it to the end! I am so proud of you. I hope you feel lighter, whole, and more aware of how amazing you are. I hope you continue to thrive, grow, and love on yourself the way you deserve to be loved on.

The great thing is this is not really the end it is only the beginning! It is a new start where you take accountability for your actions, respect others without disrespecting yourself, and love others without sacrificing so much of yourself.

There is no more shrinking, you will show up as your full self each and every time. They will either adjust or they won't... either way that is not on you.

I am so excited for you!

With Love,

Brianna Laren

P.S. Oops... I know I said this was the end but I lied (don't tell my grandma I said that word lol).

There is one more thing you need to do...

(next page)

a letter to my old self:

"I'M ROOTING FOR EVERYONE BLACK"

BLACK OWNED BUSINESSES TO ROOT FOR...

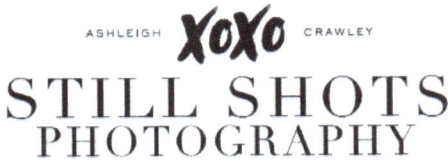
StillShotsPhotography.com

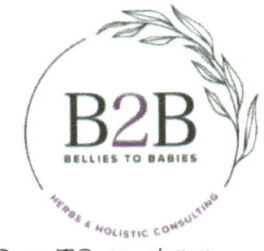
BelliesToBabiesHolistic.com

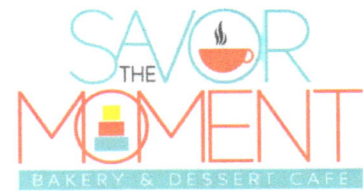
SavorTheMomentBakery.com

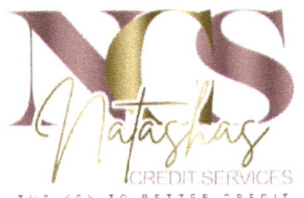
NatashasCreditServices.com

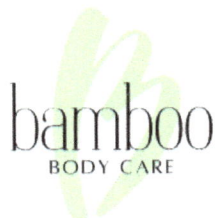
BambooBodyCare.com

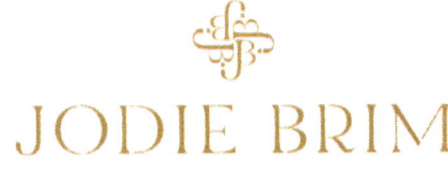
JodieBrim.com

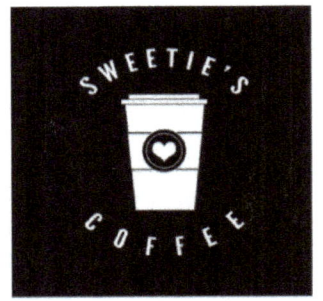
SweetiesCoffee.com

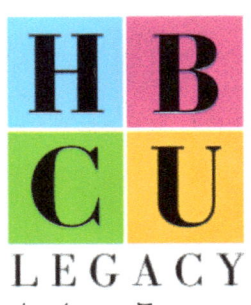
HbcuLegacyFashion.com

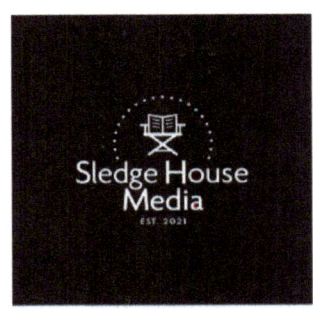
SledgeHouseMedia.com

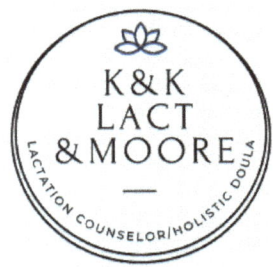
KKLactAndMoore.com

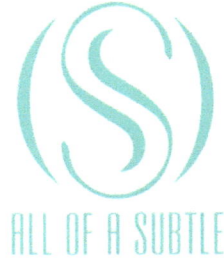
AllOfASubtle.com

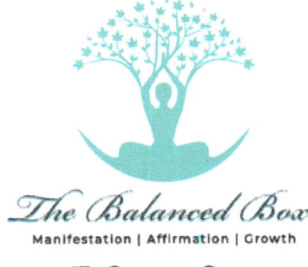
TheBalancedBox.com

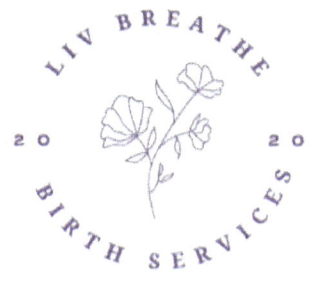
LivBreatheBirth.org

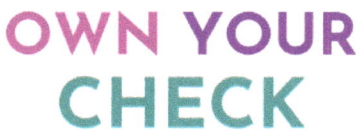
OwnYourCheck.com

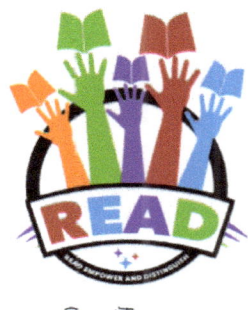
ReadInc.org

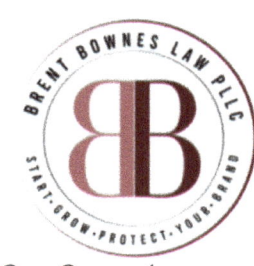
BrentBownesLaw.com

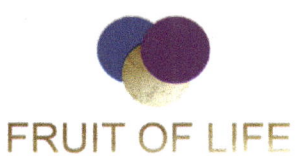
TheOGHotline.com

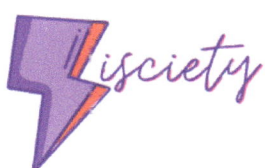
TheSisciety.com

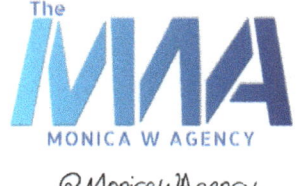
@MonicaWAgency

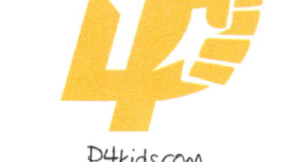
P4kids.com

Something BARowed
SomethingBARowed.com

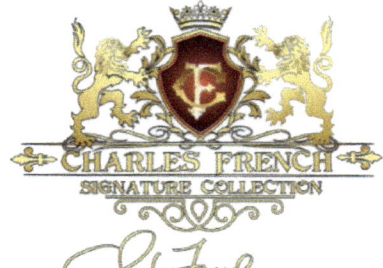
TheCharlesFrench.com

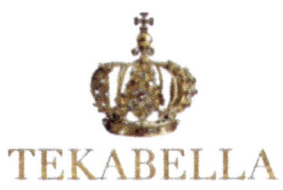
TekaBella.com

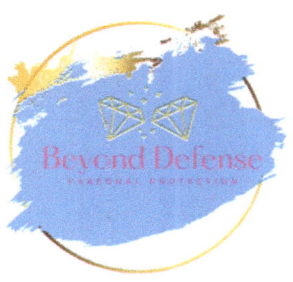
BeyondDefense.net

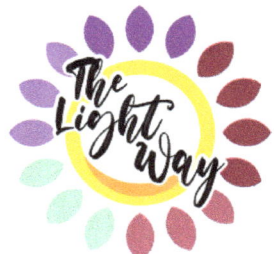
HelenHargrove.com

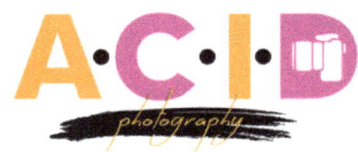
IWantAcidPhotos.square.site

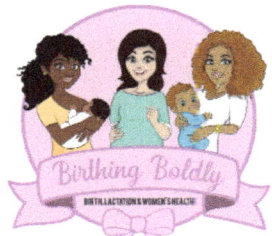
BirthingBoldlyLLC.com

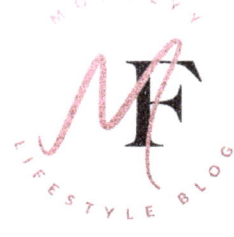
@MomFlyy

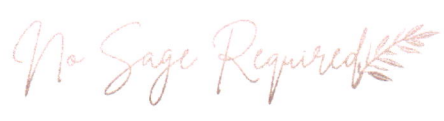
@NoSageRequired

Etsy.com/Shop/PaperbyBrandi

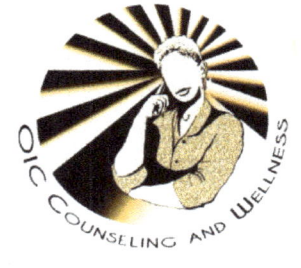
OICCounselingAndWellness.com

LETA HYCHE
REAL ESTATE

LetaHyche.com

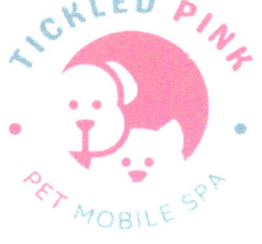
Tickled-pink-pets-mobile-spa.business.site

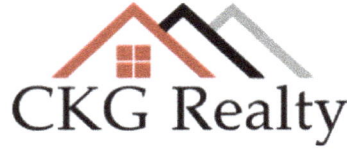
CKGRealty.com

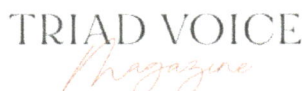
TriadVoiceMag.com

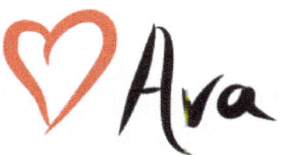
LoveAvaBoutique.com

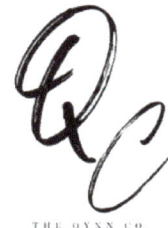
TheQynnCo.com

About The Author

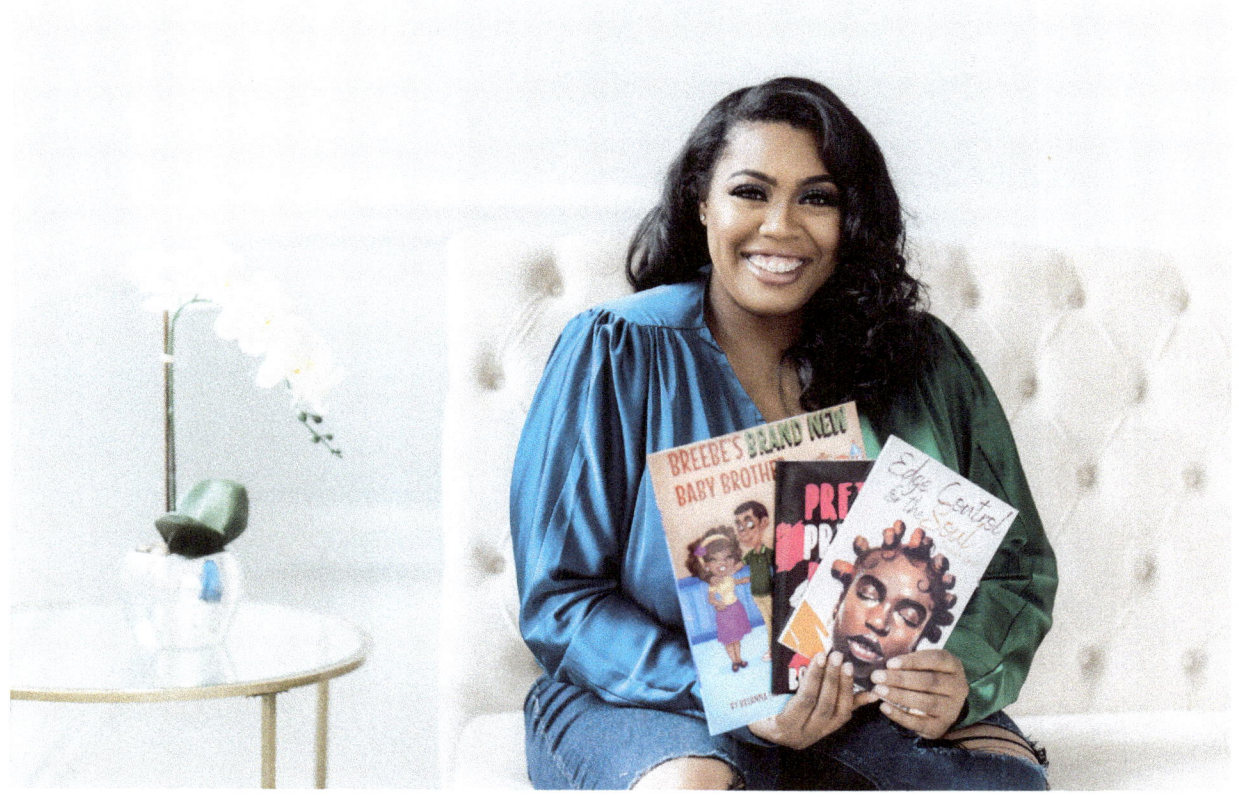

Brianna Laren is a mom, writer, and filmmaker. Born in Maryland and raised in Washington D.C, she has been writing stories, poems, and plays since she was a child, although that was mostly gibberish.

She graduated from the illustrious North Carolina A&T State University, where she received a degree in a major completely unrelated to writing. However, she attributes attending an HBCU to helping mold her into the woman she is today (making the student loan debt almost worth it).

Brianna's purpose is to create stories, characters, and content that positively reflects and uplifts the black community. Her mission is to change the narrative one keystroke at a time.

www.BriannaLaren.com | @BriannaLaren
Photo credit: Jodie Brim Photography

brain dump

www.ingramcontent.com/pod-product-compliance
Lightning Source LLC
Chambersburg PA
CBHW061805290426
44109CB00031B/2942